The Vibrant Mediterranean Dessert Collection

Quick and Easy Dessert Recipes for Getting in Shape and Boost Your Metabolism

Lexi Robertson

Table of contents

Blueberry Muffins

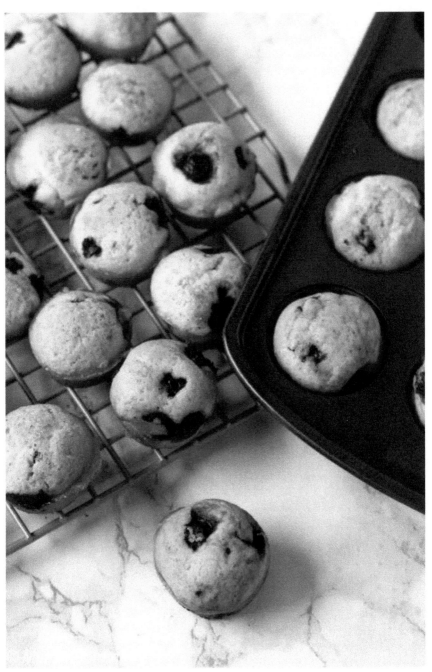

Difficulty Level: 2/5

Preparation time: 5 minutes

Cooking time: 20 mins

Servings: 24

Ingredients

2 cups all-purpose flour

2 cups whole wheat flour

2/3 cup sugar

6 teaspoons baking powder

1 teaspoon salt

2 cups blueberries

2 free-range eggs

2/3 cup olive oil

2 cups milk

Directions:

Preheat your oven to 400°F and line a muffin tin with paper cases.

Grab a large bowl and add the dry ingredients. Stir well to combine.

Add the blueberries and stir through.

Take a medium bowl and add the wet ingredients. Stir well then pour into the dry ingredients.

Pour the muffin batter into the muffin cases and pop into the oven.

Bake for 18 minutes.

Remove from the oven and allow to cool slightly before enjoying.

Nutrition: (Per serving)

Calories: 179

Net carbs: 24g

Fat: 7g

Protein: 4g

Mint Chocolate Chip Nice Cream

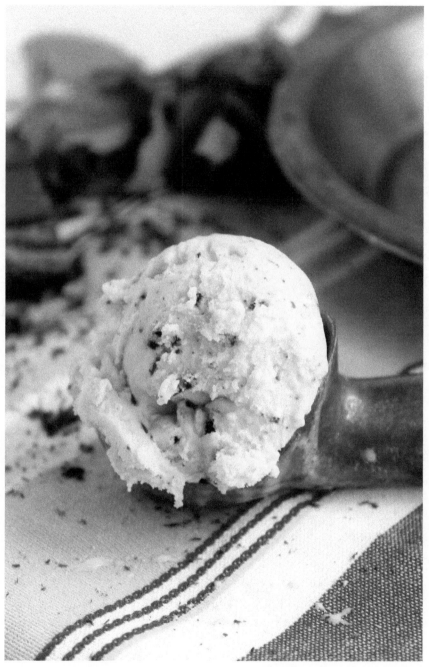

Difficulty Level: 2/5

Preparation time: 5 minutes

Cooking time: -mins

Servings: 1-2

Ingredients

2 overripe frozen bananas

Pinch salt

1/8 teaspoon pure peppermint extract

Pinch spirulina or natural food coloring (optional)

1/2 cup coconut cream

2-3 tablespoons chocolate chips

Directions:

Pop all the ingredients into your blender and whizz until smooth. Serve and enjoy.

Nutrition: (Per serving)

Calories: 601

Net carbs: 130g

Fat: 12g

Protein: 8g

Creamy Berry Crunch

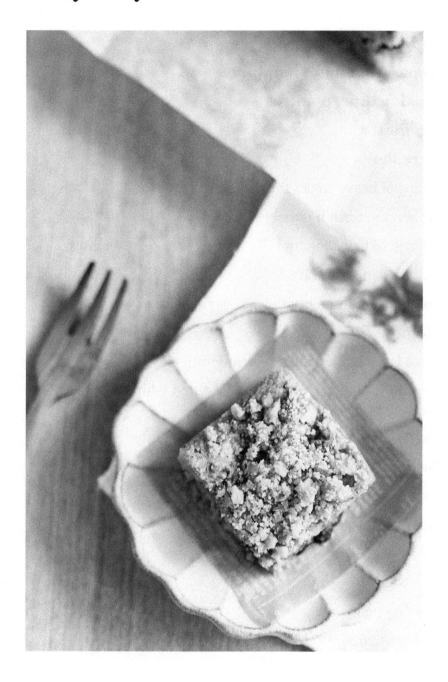

Difficulty Level: 2/5

Preparation time: 10 minutes

Cooking time: 0 mins

Servings: 2

Ingredients

2 cups of heavy cream for whipping

3oz berries, fresh if possible

The zest of half a lemon

0.25 tsp vanilla extract

2oz chopped pecan nuts

Method

Into a large bowl, whip the cream until stiff

Add the vanilla and the lemon zest and whip for a few seconds longer

Add the nuts and the berries and stir in gently

Place plastic cling film over the top of the bowl

Serve!

Nutrition

Carbs - 3g

Fat - 27g

Protein - 3g

Calories - 260

Creme Brûlée with a Gingerbread Twist

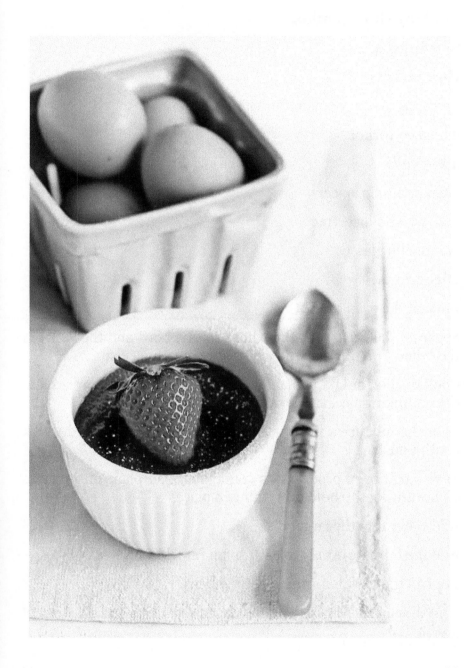

Difficulty Level: 2/5

Preparation time: 5 minutes

Cooking time: 5 mins

Servings: 4

Ingredients

1.75 cups of heavy cream for whipping

2 tbsp erythritol

4 egg yolks

2 tsp pumpkin spice

0.25 tsp vanilla extract

4 ramekin glasses

Directions:

Preheat the oven to 180C

Separate the eggs, with the whites in one bowl and the yolks in the other. You can save the whites for something else

Cook the cream in a pan and allow to boil lightly, before adding the pumpkin spice, vanilla extract and the erythritol

Pour the mixture a little at a time into the egg yolks and whisk continuously

Take small oven proof bowls (ramekins) and place into a large dish with sides to hold everything in place

Add water into the larger dish

Add the mixture evenly to each small ramekin

Cook in the oven for around half an hour

Once finished, remove the ramekins and place to one side to cool

Serve warm or cold

Nutrition

Carbs - 3g

Fat - 28g

Protein - 4g

Calories - 274

Chocolate Lava Cake

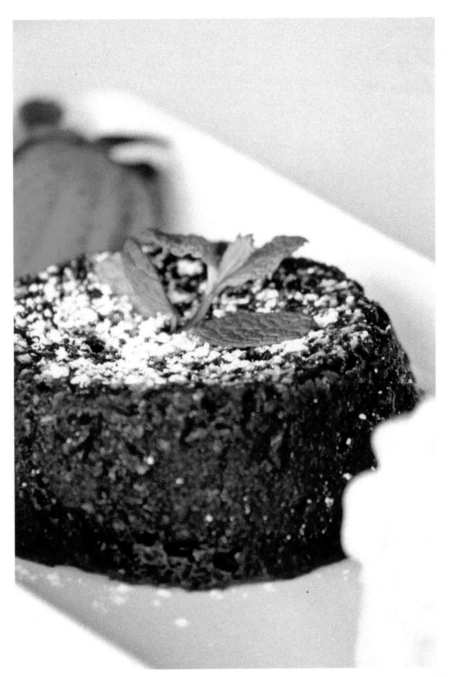

Difficulty Level: 2/5

Preparation time: 5 minutes

Cooking time: 10 mins

Serves 4

Ingredients

2oz butter

0.25 tsp vanilla extract

3 eggs

1 tbsp butter

2oz dark chocolate

4 greased ramekin glasses

Directions:

Preheat the oven to 200°C

Take four ramekin dishes and grease with butter

Cut the chocolate up into very small pieces and add to a saucepan with the butter, allowing to melt

Add the vanilla to the chocolate once melted, and stir well

Take the pan off the heat and set to one side to cool down

Crack the three eggs into a bowl and beat for around 3 minutes

Pour the chocolate mixture into the eggs and mix together well

Pour into the prepared ramekins and cook in the oven

Turn the oven down to 175°C when you place the ramekins inside, and cook for 6 minutes

Serve whilst still hot

Nutrition

Carbs - 4g

Fat - 16g

Protein - 4g

Calories - 180

Coffee Mocha Ice Cream

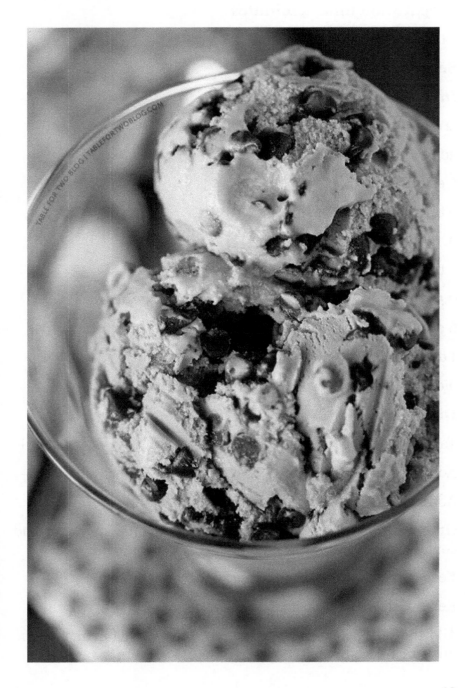

Difficulty Level: 2/5

Preparation time: 5 minutes

Cooking time: 0 mins

Serves 4

Ingredients

2 cups of heavy cream for whipping

3oz chopped dark chocolate

6 egg yolks

2 tbsp coffee powder (instant)

0.75 cup of erythritol powder

2 tsp vanilla extract

0.5 tsp salt

6 drops of liquid sweetener

1 drop of peppermint extract

For this recipe you will need an ice cream maker

Directions:

Take a large saucepan and warm up the cream, stirring constantly

Add the dark chocolate and keep stirring until it has all melted

Add the egg yolks into the pan and stir constantly

Once warm, add the erythritol powder, coffee powder, and combine well

Keep stirring until a custard consistency is achieved

Remove the pan and place to one side

Add the salt, peppermint extract, and the vanilla extract to the mixture and combine

Add the liquid sweetener and combine once more

Place the pan into the refrigerator to cool completely

Transfer the mixture into the ice cream maker and follow the instructions to create delicious ice cream.

Nutrition

Carbs - 5g

Fat - 40g

Protein - 7g

Calories - 422

Chocolate & Pecan Thins

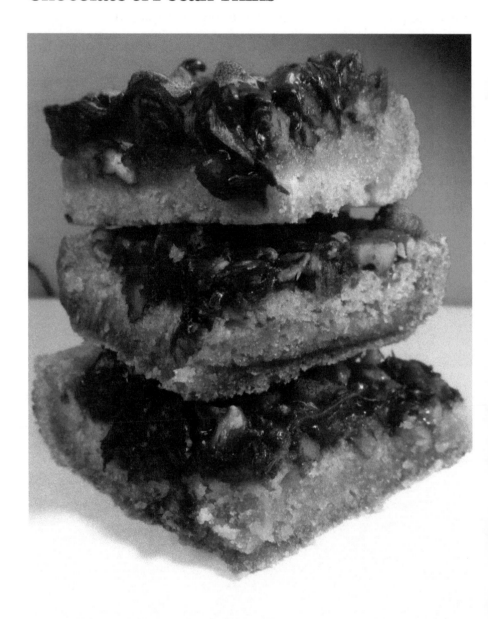

Difficulty Level: 2/5

Preparation time: 5 minutes

Cooking time: 10 mins

Serves 4

Ingredients

4oz dark chocolate

0.5oz pecans, chopped

0.25 tsp vanilla extract

1 tsp liquorice powder

Baking tray lined with parchment paper

Directions:

Warm up a pan on a low heat and melt the chocolate, or place in the microwave as an alternative

Add the liquorice and the vanilla extract and combine well

Take a baking tray and grease it, lining it with parchment paper

Pour the mixture onto the tray and add the pecans over the top

Allow to cool or place in the refrigerator if you want it faster!

The mixture should set to a completely hard consistency - snap to break up, to around 15 pieces and enjoy!

Nutrition

Carbs - 3g

Fat - 5g

Protein - 1g

Calories - 60

Banana Blue Berry Blast

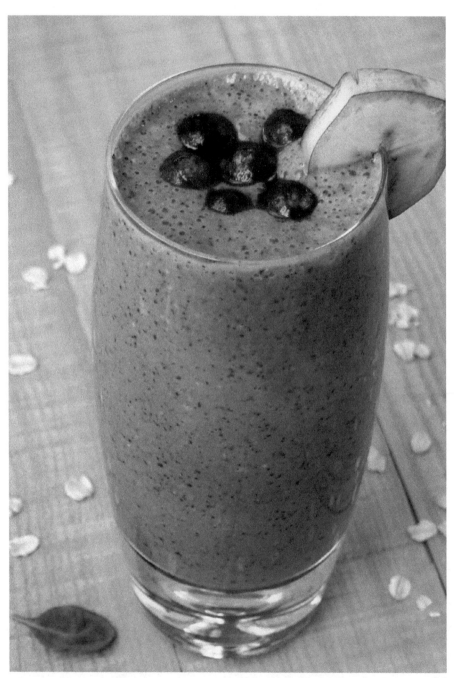

Difficulty Level: 2/5

Preparation time: 4 minutes

Cooking time: None

Servings:: 2

Ingredients:

½ cup oats

1 ½ cups plain nonfat Greek yogurt

1 cup blueberries

1 banana

5 walnuts

Directions:

Add all the ingredients to a blender and blend until very smooth. Enjoy!

Nutrition:

Calories: 300

Carbohydrates: 22.5 g

Fats: 4 g

Proteins: 5 g

Pistachio and Fruits

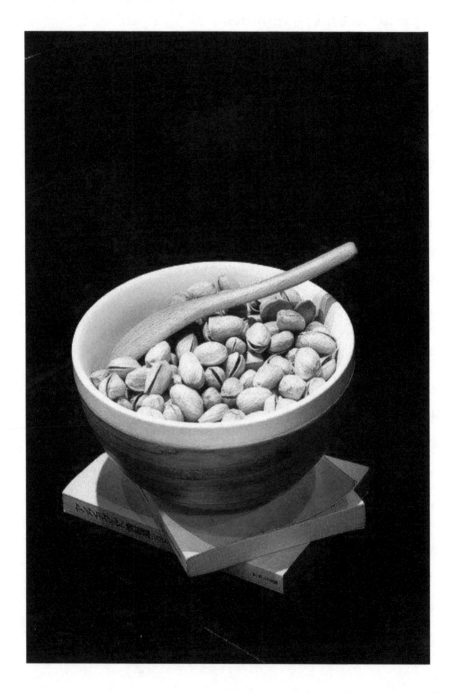

Difficulty Level: 2/5

Preparation time: 5 minutes

Cooking time: 7 minutes

Servings: 12

Ingredients:

½ cup apricots, dried and chopped

¼ cup dried cranberries

½ tsp. cinnamon

¼ tsp. allspice

¼ tsp. ground nutmeg

1 ¼ cups unsalted pistachios, roasted

2 tsp. sugar

Directions:

Start by heating the oven to a temperature of around 345 degrees F.

Using a tray, place the pistachios and bake for seven minutes. Allow the pistachio to cool afterward.

Combine all ingredients on a container.

Once everything is combined well the food is ready to serve.

Nutrition:

Calories: 377

Carbohydrates: 24.5 g

Fats: 5 g

Proteins: 16 g

Avocado Sorbet

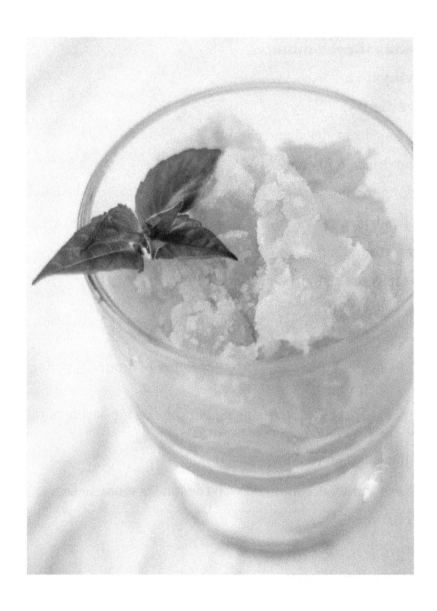

Difficulty Level: 2/5

Preparation time: 5 minutes

Cooking time: 10 minutes

Servings: 4

Ingredients:

¼ cup of sugar

1 cup of water

1 tsp grated lime zest

1 tbsp honey

2 ripe avocados, pitted and skin removed

2 tbsp lime juice

Directions:

Combine together the sugar and water in a small pan over medium flame. Continue until the sugar dissolves completely and then remove from the flame.

Place the avocados in the food processor. Add the sugar and water mix along with the honey, lime zest, and lime juice into the food processor.

Process until you reach a smooth consistency.

Place the mix into a baking pan and cover with foil. Place the mix into the freezer until completely frozen.

Upon serving, process the food in the food processor until you reach a smooth consistency.

Nutrition:

Calories: 390.3 | Carbohydrates: 19 g

Fats: 6 g | Proteins: 10 g

Cioccolata Calda

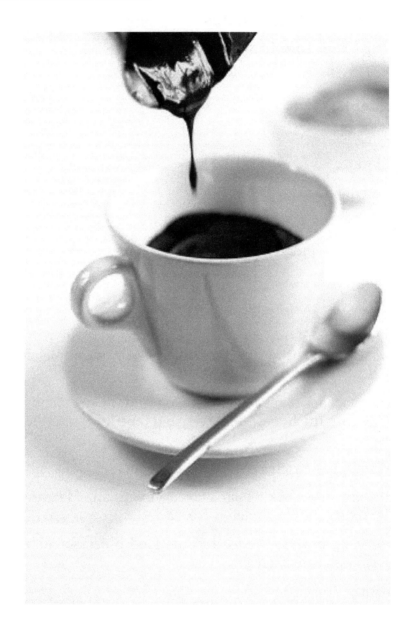

Difficulty Level: 2/5

Preparation time: 5 minutes

Cooking time: 10 minutes

Servings: 2

Ingredients:

1½ tbsp sugar

1 tbsp cornstarch

3 tbsp unsweetened cocoa powder

1½ cups plus 2 tbsp milk

Directions:

Mix together the cocoa powder and sugar in a little frying pan. Add one and a half cups of milk while mixing. Start with medium heat and gradually lower until the sugar is fully dissolved. The entire mixture should simmer.

In a separate container, mix the cornstarch and the remaining two tablespoons of milk. After being mixed add to the cocoa mix on the frying pan.

Continue mixing until the entire mixture reaches a thick consistency. Serve while hot.

Nutrition:

Calories: 427 | Carbohydrates: 22 g

Fats: 4 g | Proteins: 12 g

Maple Brown Rice Pudding

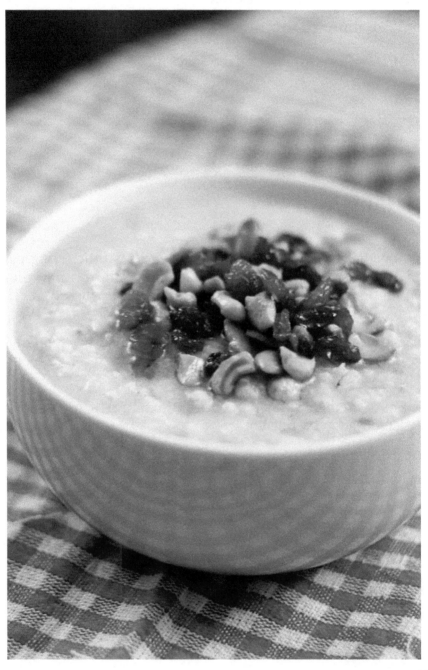

Difficulty Level: 2/5

Preparation time: 5 minutes

Cooking time: 15 minutes

Servings: 8

Ingredients:

½ cup packed light brown sugar

¼ cup pure maple syrup

½ tsp ground cinnamon

¼ tsp ground nutmeg

pinch of salt

1 tsp vanilla extract

2 cups cooked brown rice

3 cups unsweetened almond milk

3 eggs

Directions:

Place the entire ingredients into a large container and mix well.

Using a spoon, place the mixture into oil-coated microwave-safe plates (five to six plates).

Cook the mixture in the microwave for two minutes.

Place the puddings into one single bowl and serve.

Nutrition:

Calories: 320

Carbohydrates: 23 g

Fats: 8 g

Proteins: 8 g

Raspberry Curd

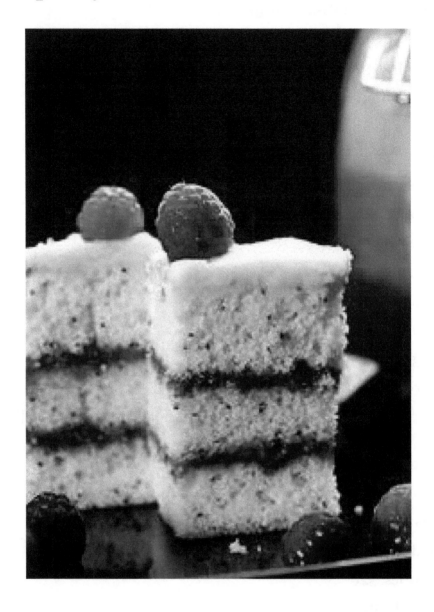

Difficulty Level: 2/5

Preparation time: 10 minutes

Cooking time: 5 minutes

Servings: 4

Ingredients:

1 cup sugar

12 ounces raspberries

2 egg yolks

2 tablespoons lemon juice

2 tablespoons butter

Directions:

Put the raspberries into the Pressure Pot. Add the sugar and lemon juice, stir, cover, and cook on the Manual setting for 2 minutes.

Release the pressure for 5 minutes, uncover the Pressure Pot, strain the raspberries and discard the seeds.

In a bowl, mix the egg yolks with raspberries and stir well. Return this to the Pressure Pot, set it on Sauté mode, simmer for 2 minutes, add the butter, stir, and transfer to a container. Serve cold.

Nutrition:

Calories: 110

Fat: 4

Fiber: 0

Carbs: 16

Protein: 1

Pear Jam

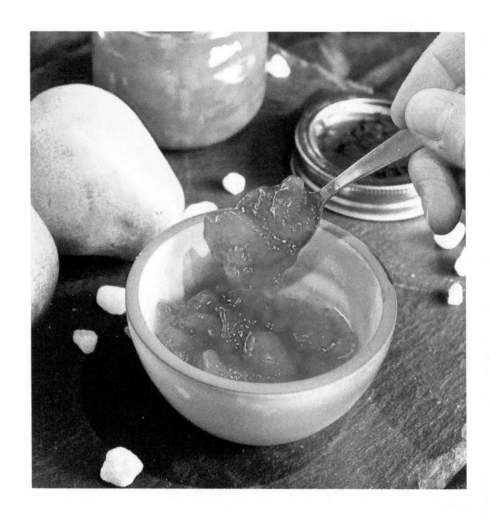

Difficulty Level: 2/5

Preparation time: 10 minutes

Cooking time: 4 minutes

Servings: 12

Ingredients:

8 pears, cored and cut into quarters

2 apples, peeled, cored, and cut into quarters

¼ cup apple juice

1 teaspoon cinnamon, ground

Directions:

In the Pressure Pot, mix the pears with apples, cinnamon, and apple juice, stir, cover, and cook on the Manual setting for 4 minutes. Release the pressure naturally, uncover the Pressure Pot, blend using an immersion blender, divide the jam into jars, and keep in a cold place until you serve it.

Nutrition:

Calories: 90

Fat: 0

Fiber: 1

Carbs: 20

Sugar: 20

Protein: 0

Berry Compote

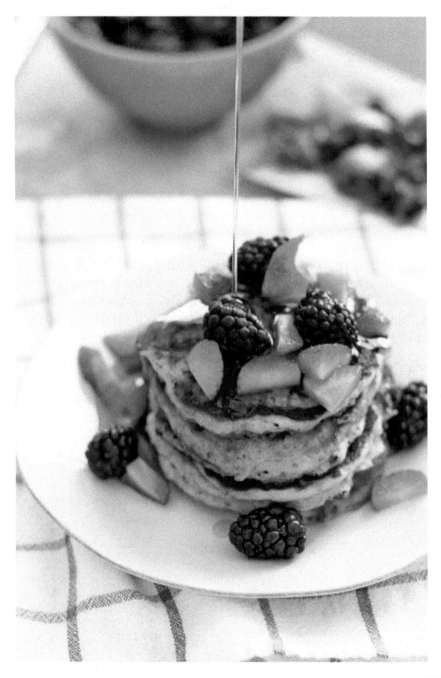

Difficulty Level: 2/5

Preparation time: 10 minutes

Cooking time: 5 minutes

Servings: 8

Ingredients:

1 cup blueberries

2 cups strawberries, sliced

2 tablespoons lemon juice

¾ cup sugar

1 tablespoon cornstarch

1 tablespoon water

Directions:

In the Pressure Pot, mix the blueberries with lemon juice and sugar, stir, cover, and cook on the Manual setting for 3 minutes. Release the pressure naturally for 10 minutes and uncover the Pressure Pot. In a bowl, mix the cornstarch with water, stir well, and add to the Pressure Pot. Stir, set the Pressure Pot on Sauté mode, and cook compote for 2 minutes. Divide into jars and keep in the refrigerator until you serve it.

Nutrition:

Calories: 260

Fat: 13

Fiber: 3

Carbs: 23

Protein: 3

Key Lime Pie

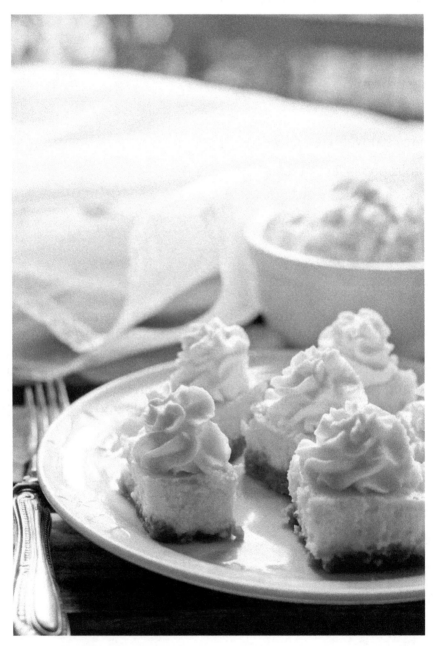

Difficulty Level: 2/5

Preparation time: 10 minutes

Cooking time: 15 minutes

Servings: 6

Ingredients:

For the crust:

1 tablespoon sugar

3 tablespoons butter, melted

5 graham crackers, crumbled

For the filling:

4 egg yolks

14 ounces canned condensed milk

½ cup key lime juice

⅓ cup sour cream

Vegetable oil cooking spray

1 cup water

2 tablespoons key lime zest, grated

Directions:

In a bowl, whisk the egg yolks well. Add the milk gradually and stir again. Add the lime juice, sour cream, and lime zest and stir again. In another bowl, whisk the butter with the graham crackers and sugar, stir well, and spread on the bottom of a spring form greased with some cooking spray. Cover the pan with some aluminum foil and place it in the steamer basket of the Pressure Pot. Add the water to the Pressure Pot, cover and cook on the Manual setting for 15 minutes. Release the pressure for 10 minutes, uncover the Pressure Pot, take the pie out, set aside to cool down and keep in the refrigerator for 4 hours before slicing and serving it.

Nutrition:

Calories: 400

Fat: 21

Fiber: 0.5

Carbs: 34

Protein: 7

Fruit Cobbler

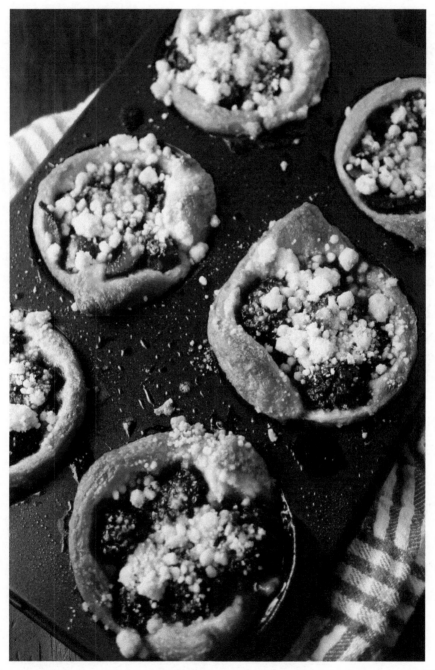

Difficulty Level: 2/5

Preparation time: 10 minutes

Cooking time: 12 minutes

Servings: 4

Ingredients:

3 apples, cored and cut into chunks

2 pears, cored and cut into chunks

1½ cup hot water

¼ cup honey

1 cup steel-cut oats

1 teaspoon ground cinnamon

ice cream, for serving

Directions:

Put the apples and pears into the Pressure Pot and mix with hot water, honey, oats, and cinnamon. Stir, cover, and cook on the Manual setting for 12 minutes. Release the pressure naturally, transfer

Nutrition:

Calories: 170

Fat: 4

Carbs: 10

Fiber: 2.4

Protein: 3

Sugar: 7

Stuffed Peaches

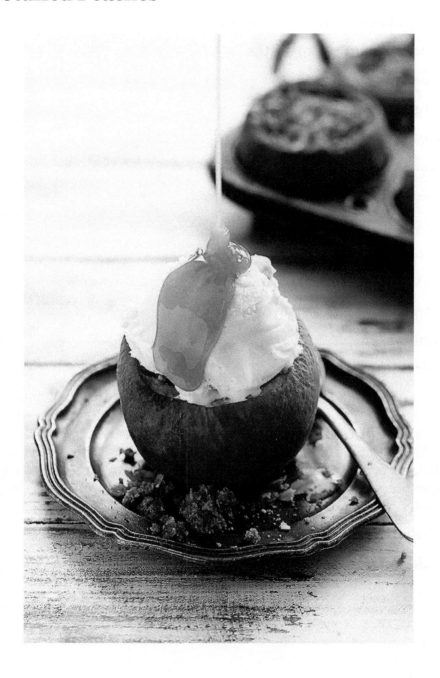

Difficulty Level: 2/5

Preparation time: 10 minutes

Cooking time: 4 minutes

Servings: 6

Ingredients:

6 peaches, pits and flesh removed

Salt

¼ cup coconut flour

¼ cup maple syrup

2 tablespoons coconut butter

½ teaspoon ground cinnamon

1 teaspoon almond extract

1 cup water

Directions:

In a bowl, mix the flour with the salt, syrup, butter, cinnamon, and half of the almond extract and stir well. Fill the peaches with this mix, place them in the steamer basket of the Pressure Pot, add the water and the rest of the almond extract to the Pressure Pot, cover and cook on the Steam setting for 4 minutes. Release the pressure naturally, divide the stuffed peaches on serving plates, and serve warm.

Nutrition:

Calories: 160

Fat: 6.7

Carbs: 12

Fiber: 3

Sugar: 11

Protein: 4

Peach Compote

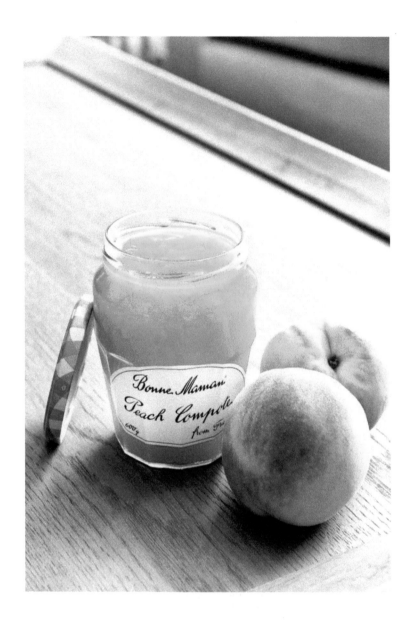

Difficulty Level: 2/5

Preparation time: 10 minutes

Cooking time: 3 minutes

Servings: 6

Ingredients:

8 peaches, pitted and chopped

6 tablespoons sugar

1 teaspoon ground cinnamon

1 teaspoon vanilla extract

1 vanilla bean, scraped

2 tablespoons Grape Nuts cereal

Directions:

Put the peaches into the Pressure Pot and mix with the sugar, cinnamon, vanilla bean, and vanilla extract. Stir well, cover the Pressure Pot and cook on the Manual setting for 3 minutes. Release the pressure for 10 minutes, add the cereal, stir well, transfer the compote to bowls, and serve.

Nutrition:

Calories: 100

Fat: 2

Carbs: 11

Fiber: 1

Sugar: 10

Protein: 1

Chocolate Pudding

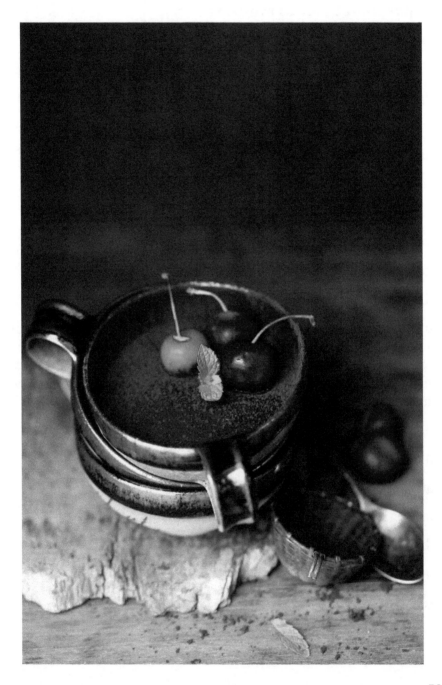

Difficulty Level: 2/5

Preparation time: 10 minutes

Cooking time: 20 minutes

Servings: 4

Ingredients:

6 ounces bittersweet chocolate, chopped

½ cup milk

1½ cups heavy cream

5 egg yolks

⅓ cup brown sugar

2 teaspoons vanilla extract

1½ cups water

¼ teaspoon cardamom

Salt

Crème fraîche, for serving

Chocolate shavings, for serving

Directions:

Put the cream and milk in a pot, bring to a simmer over medium heat, take off the heat, add the chocolate and whisk well. In a bowl, mix the egg yolks with the vanilla, sugar, cardamom, and a pinch of salt, stir, strain, and mix with chocolate mixture. Pour this into a soufflé dish, cover with aluminum foil, place in the steamer basket of the Pressure Pot, add water to the Pressure Pot, cover, cook on Manual for 18 minutes, release the pressure naturally.

Take the pudding out of the Pressure Pot, set aside to cool down and keep it in the refrigerator for 3 hours before serving with crème fraîche and chocolate shavings on top.

Nutrition:

Calories: 200

Fat: 3

Fiber: 1

Carbs: 20

Protein: 14

Refreshing Curd

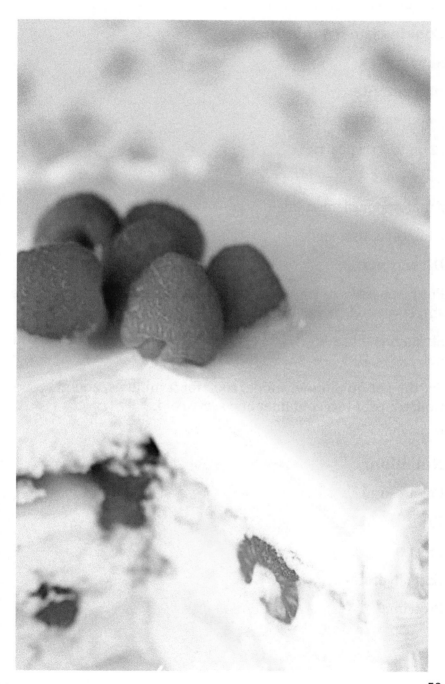

Difficulty Level: 2/5

Preparation time: 10 minutes

Cooking time: 5 minutes

Servings: 4

Ingredients:

3 tablespoons stevia

12 ounces raspberries

2 egg yolks

2 tablespoons lemon juice

2 tablespoons ghee

Directions:

Put raspberries in your Pressure Pot, add stevia and lemon juice, stir, cover and cook on High for 2 minutes.

Strain this into a bowl, add egg yolks, stir well and return to your pot.

Set the pot on Simmer mode, cook for 2 minutes, add ghee, stir well, transfer to a container and serve cold.

Enjoy!

Nutrition:

Calories 132,

Fat 1,

Fiber 0,

Carbohydrates 2,

Protein 4

The Best Jam Ever

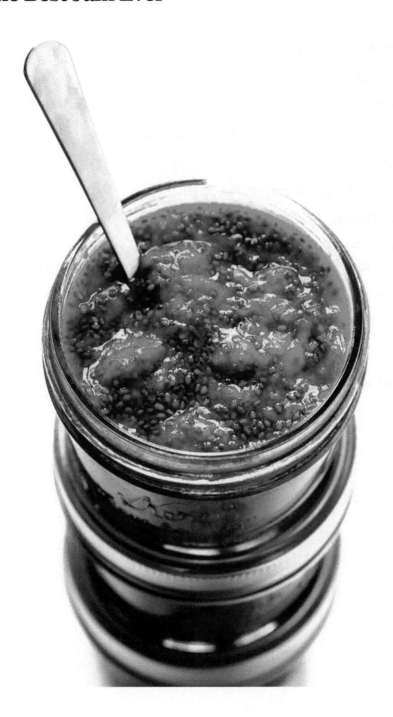

Difficulty Level: 2/5

Preparation time: 10 minutes

Cooking time: 5 minutes

Servings: 6

Ingredients:

4 and ½ cups peaches, peeled and cubed

4 tablespoons stevia

¼ cup crystallized ginger, chopped

Directions:

Set your Pressure Pot on Simmer mode, add peaches, ginger and stevia, stir, bring to a boil, cover and cook on High for 5 minutes.

Divide into bowls and serve cold.

Enjoy!

Nutrition:

Calories 53,

Fat 0,

Fiber 0,

Carbs 0,

Protein 2g

Divine Pears

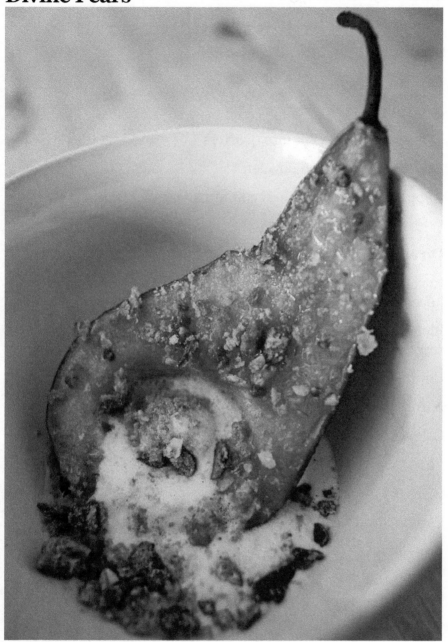

Difficulty Level: 2/5

Preparation time: 10 minutes

Cooking time: 4 minutes

Servings: 12

Ingredients:

8 pears, cored and cut into quarters

1 teaspoon cinnamon powder

2 apples, peeled, cored and cut into quarters

¼ cup natural apple juice

Directions:

In your Pressure Pot, mix pears with apples, cinnamon and apple juice, stir, cover and cook on High for 4 minutes.

Blend using an immersion blender, divide into small jars and serve cold

Enjoy!

Nutrition:

Calories 100,

Fat 0,

Fiber 0,

Carbohydrates 0,

Protein 2g

Chocolate Pudding in a Mug

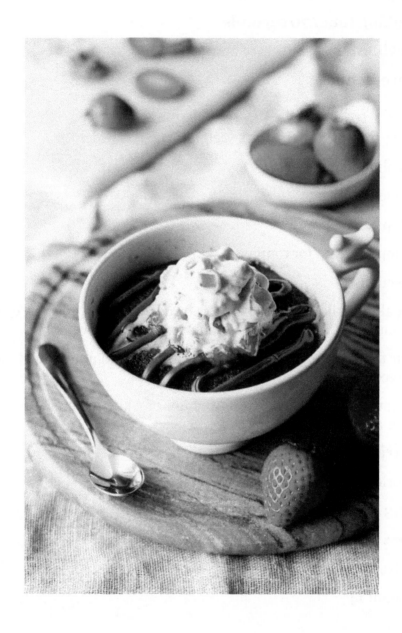

Difficulty Level: 2/5

Preparation time: 10 minutes

Cooking time: 70 seconds

Servings: 2

Ingredients:

2 eggs oz almond

Flour tbsp xylitol tbsp unsweetened cocoa powder

1 oz almond milk

Tbsp olive oil

½ tsp baking powder

Whipped cream for topping

Directions

Mix almond flour, xylitol, cocoa powder, espresso powder, eggs, coconut milk, olive oil, and baking powder in a bowl.

Pour the mix into mugs ¾ way up and cook in a microwave for 70 seconds.

Remove and swirl a generous amount of whipping cream on the cakes and serve.

Nutrition:

Calories: 200

Fat: 3

Fiber: 1

Carbs: 20

Protein: 14

Healthy Fruit Salad with Yogurt Cream

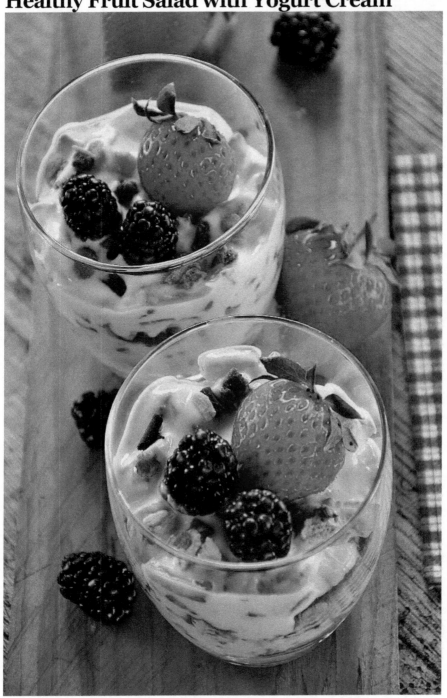

Difficulty Level: 2/5

Preparation time: 10 minutes

Cooking time: 0 minutes

Servings: 4

Ingredients:

1 1/2 cups grapes halved

2 plums chopped

1 peach chopped

1 cup chopped cantaloupe

1/2 cup fresh blueberries

1 cup unsweetened plain nonfat Greek yogurt

1/2 teaspoon ground cinnamon

2 tablespoons honey

Directions:

In a large bowl combine the grapes plums peach cantaloupe and blueberries. Toss to mix. Divide among 4 dessert dishes.

In a small bowl whisk the yogurt ,cinnamon and honey. Spoon over the fruit.

Sprinkle yogurt with sugar and drizzle with honey. Serve fruit with yogurt mixture.

Nutrition

Calories (Per Serving): 74

Fat: 0.7g

Carbohydrates: 16g

Protein: 2g

Summertime Fruit Salad

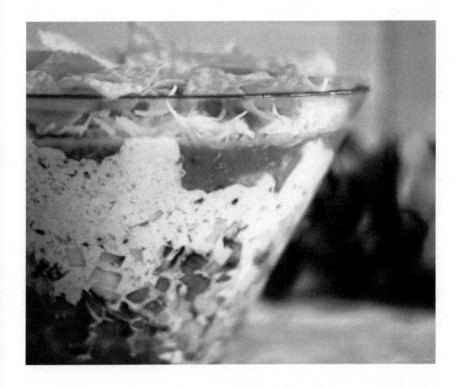

Difficulty Level: 2/5

Cooking Time: 0 minutes

Preparation time: 30 minutes

Servings: 6

Ingredients:

1-pound strawberries, hulled and sliced thinly

3 medium peaches, sliced thinly

6 ounces blueberries

1 tablespoon fresh mint, chopped

2 tablespoons lemon juice

1 tablespoon honey

2 teaspoons balsamic vinegar

Directions:

In a salad bowl, combine all ingredients.

Gently toss to coat all ingredients.

Chill for at least 30 minutes before serving.

Nutrition:

Calories per serving: 146;

Carbs: 22.8g;

Protein: 8.1g;

Fat: 3.4g

Banana Shake Bowls

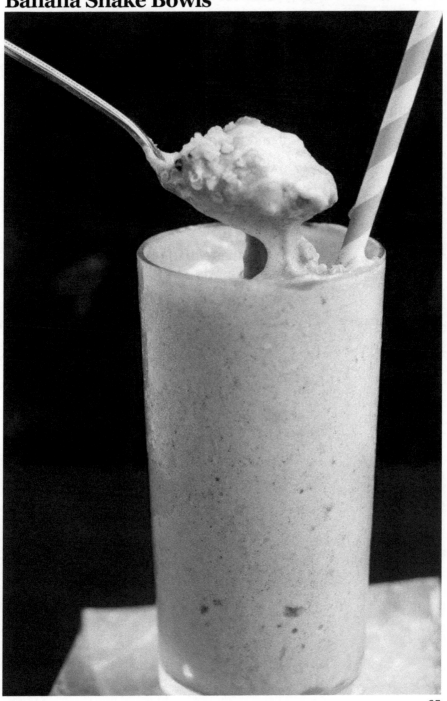

Preparation Time: 5 minutes

Cooking Time: 0 minutes

Servings: 4

Ingredients:

4 medium bananas, peeled

1 avocado, peeled, pitted and mashed

¾ cup almond milk

½ teaspoon vanilla extract

Directions:

In a blender, combine the bananas with the avocado and the other ingredients, pulse, divide into bowls and keep in the fridge until serving.

Nutrition:

Calories 185

Fat 4.3

Fiber 4

Carbs 6

Protein 6.45

Cold Lemon Squares

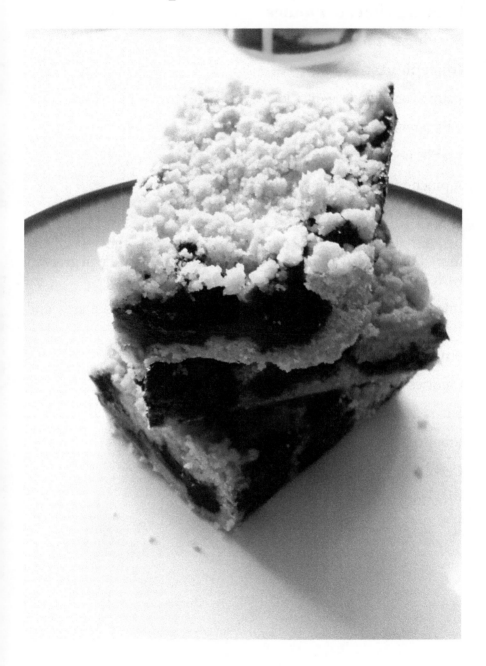

Preparation Time: 30 minutes

Cooking Time: 0 minutes

Servings: 4

Ingredients:

1 cup avocado oil+ a drizzle

2 bananas, peeled and chopped

1 tablespoon honey ¼ cup lemon juice

A pinch of lemon zest, grated

Directions:

In your food processor, mix the bananas with the rest of the ingredients, pulse well and spread on the bottom of a pan greased with a drizzle of oil.

Introduce in the fridge for 30 minutes, slice into squares and serve.

Nutrition:

Calories 136

Fat 11.2

Fiber 0.2

Carbs 7

Protein 1.1

Strawberries Cream

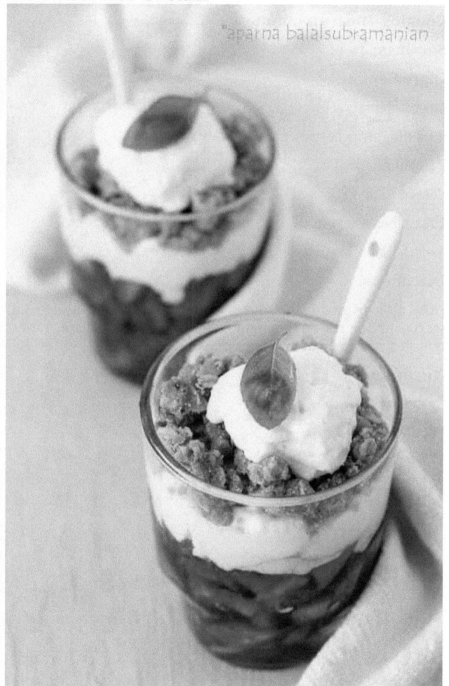

aparna balalsubramanian

Preparation Time: 10 minutes

Cooking Time: 20 minutes

Servings: 4

Ingredients:

½ cup stevia

2 pounds strawberries, chopped

1 cup almond milk

Zest of 1 lemon, grated

½ cup heavy cream

3 egg yolks, whisked

Directions:

Heat up a pan with the milk over medium-high heat, add the stevia and the rest of the ingredients, whisk well, simmer for 20 minutes, divide into cups and serve cold.

Nutrition:

Calories 152

Fat 4.4

Fiber 5.5

Carbs 5.1

Protein 0.8

Cinnamon Chickpeas Cookies

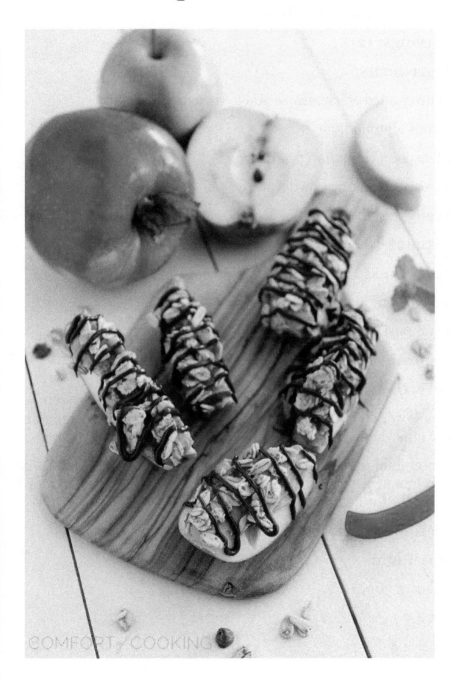

Preparation Time: 10 minutes

Cooking Time: 20 minutes

Servings: 12

Ingredients:

1 cup canned chickpeas, drained, rinsed and mashed

2 cups almond flour

1 teaspoon cinnamon powder

1 teaspoon baking powder

1 cup avocado oil

½ cup stevia

1 egg, whisked

2 teaspoons almond extract

1 cup raisins

1 cup coconut, unsweetened and shredded

Directions:

In a bowl, combine the chickpeas with the flour, cinnamon and the other ingredients, and whisk well until you obtain a dough.

Scoop tablespoons of dough on a baking sheet lined with parchment paper, introduce them in the oven at 350 degrees F and bake for 20 minutes.

Leave them to cool down for a few minutes and serve.

Nutrition:

Calories 200

Fat 4.5

Fiber 3.4

Carbs 9.5

Protein 2.4

Cocoa Brownies

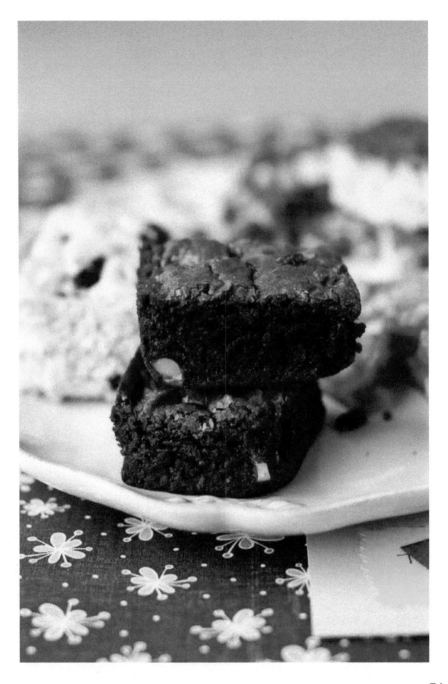

Preparation Time: 10 minutes

Cooking Time: 20 minutes

Servings: 8

Ingredients:

30 ounces canned lentils, rinsed and drained

1 tablespoon honey

1 banana, peeled and chopped

½ teaspoon baking soda

4 tablespoons almond butter

2 tablespoons cocoa powder

Cooking spray

Directions:

In a food processor, combine the lentils with the honey and the other ingredients except the cooking spray and pulse well.

Pour this into a pan greased with cooking spray, spread evenly, introduce in the oven at 375 degrees F and bake for 20 minutes.

Cut the brownies and serve cold.

Nutrition:

Calories 200

Fat 4.5

Fiber 2.4

Carbs 8.7

Protein 4.3

Cardamom Almond Cream

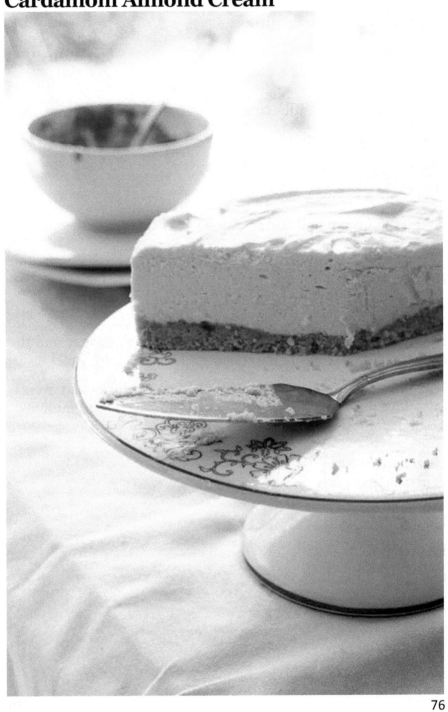

Preparation Time: 30 minutes

Cooking Time: 0 minutes

Servings: 4

Ingredients:

Juice of 1 lime

½ cup stevia

1 and ½ cups water

3 cups almond milk

½ cup honey

2 teaspoons cardamom, ground

1 teaspoon rose water

1 teaspoon vanilla extract

Directions:

In a blender, combine the almond milk with the cardamom and the rest of the ingredients, pulse well, divide into cups and keep in the fridge for 30 minutes before serving.

Nutrition:

Calories 283

Fat 11.8

Fiber 0.3

Carbs

Protein 7.1

Banana Cinnamon Cupcakes

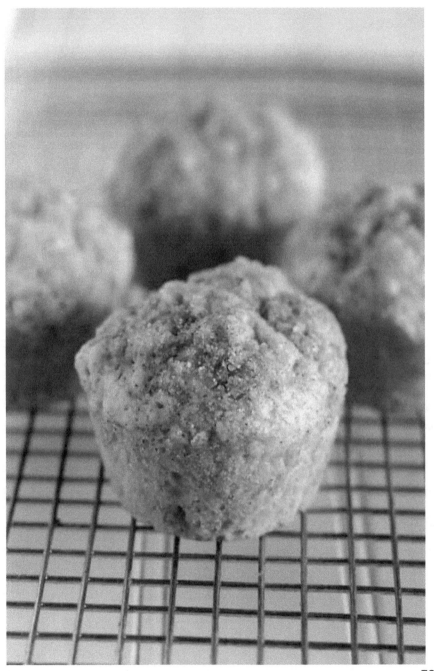

Preparation Time: 10 minutes

Cooking Time: 20 minutes

Servings: 4

Ingredients:

4 tablespoons avocado oil

4 eggs

½ cup orange juice

2 teaspoons cinnamon powder

1 teaspoon vanilla extract

2 bananas, peeled and chopped

¾ cup almond flour

½ teaspoon baking powder

Cooking spray

Directions:

In a bowl, combine the oil with the eggs, orange juice and the other ingredients except the cooking spray, whisk well, pour in a cupcake pan greased with the cooking spray, introduce in the oven at 350 degrees F and bake for 20 minutes.

Cool the cupcakes down and serve.

Nutrition:

Calories 142

Fat 5.8

Fiber 4.2

Carbs 5.7

Protein 1.6

Rhubarb and Apples Cream

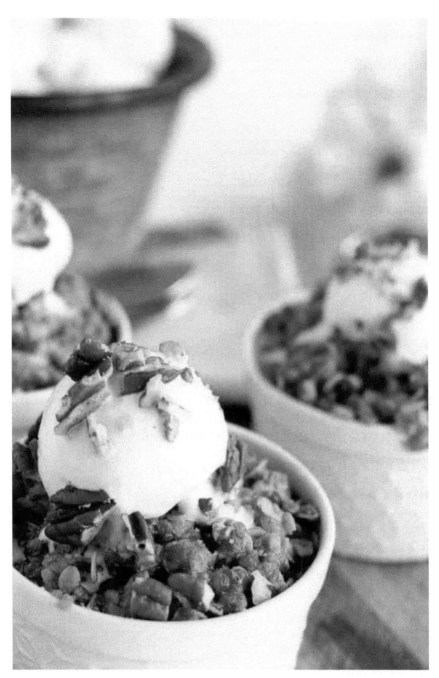

Preparation Time: 10 minutes

Cooking Time: 0 minutes

Servings: 6

Ingredients:

3 cups rhubarb, chopped

1 and ½ cups stevia

2 eggs, whisked

½ teaspoon nutmeg, ground

1 tablespoon avocado oil

1/3 cup almond milk

Directions:

In a blender, combine the rhubarb with the stevia and the rest of the ingredients, pulse well, divide into cups and serve cold.

Nutrition:

Calories 200

Fat 5.2

Fiber 3.4

Carbs 7.6

Protein 2.5

Almond Rice Dessert

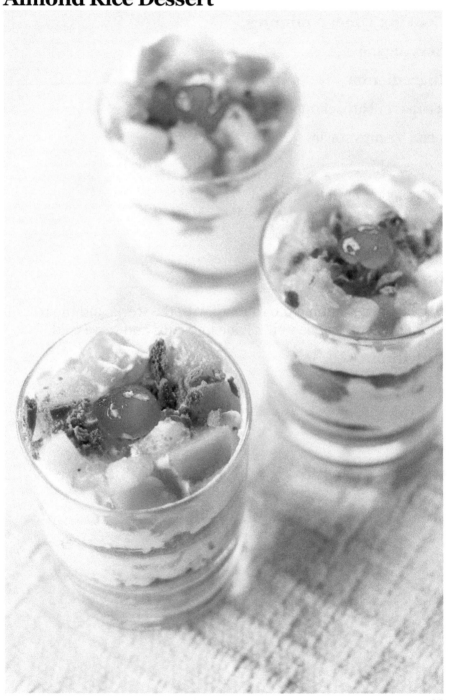

Preparation Time: 10 minutes

Cooking Time: 20 minutes

Servings: 4

Ingredients:

1 cup white rice

2 cups almond milk

1 cup almonds, chopped

½ cup stevia

1 tablespoon cinnamon powder

½ cup pomegranate seeds

Directions:

In a pot, mix the rice with the milk and stevia, bring to a simmer and cook for 20 minutes, stirring often.

Add the rest of the ingredients, stir, divide into bowls and serve.

Nutrition:

Calories 234

Fat 9.5

Fiber 3.4

Carbs 12.4

Protein 6.5

Blueberries Stew

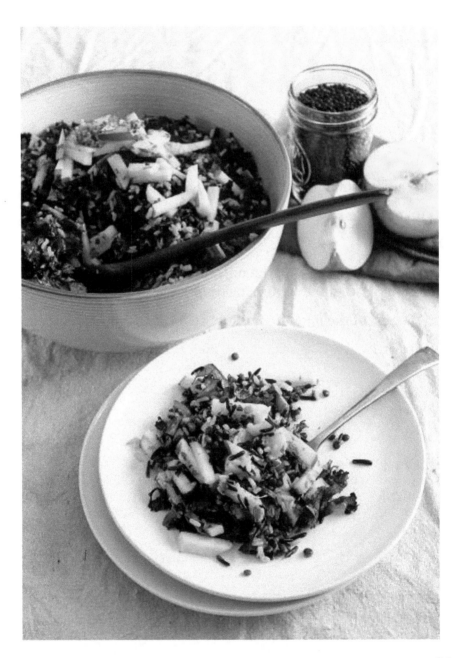

Preparation Time: 10 minutes

Cooking Time: 10 minutes

Servings: 4

Ingredients:

2 cups blueberries

3 tablespoons stevia

1 and ½ cups pure apple juice

1 teaspoon vanilla extract

Directions:

In a pan, combine the blueberries with stevia and the other ingredients, bring to a simmer and cook over medium-low heat for 10 minutes.

Divide into cups and serve cold.

Nutrition:

Calories 192

Fat 5.4

Fiber 3.4

Carbs 9.4

Protein 4.5

Mandarin Cream

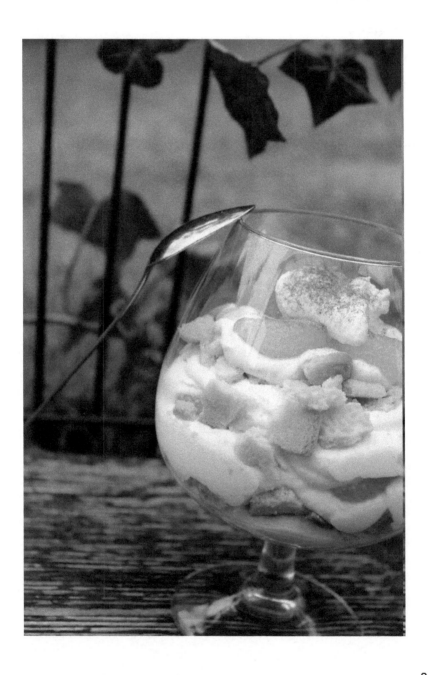

Preparation Time: 20 minutes

Cooking Time: 0 minutes

Servings: 8

Ingredients:

2 mandarins, peeled and cut into segments

Juice of 2 mandarins

2 tablespoons stevia

4 eggs, whisked

¾ cup stevia

¾ cup almonds, ground

Directions:

In a blender, combine the mandarins with the mandarins juice and the other ingredients, whisk well, divide into cups and keep in the fridge for 20 minutes before serving.

Nutrition:

Calories 106

Fat 3.4

Fiber 0

Carbs 2.4

Protein 4

Pumpkin Cream

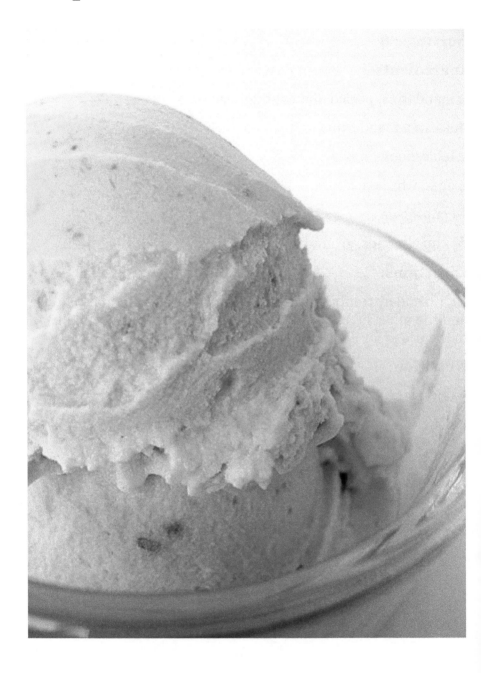

Preparation Time: 5 minutes

Cooking Time: 5 minutes

Servings: 2

Ingredients:

2 cups canned pumpkin flesh

2 tablespoons stevia

1 teaspoon vanilla extract

2 tablespoons water

A pinch of pumpkin spice

Directions:

In a pan, combine the pumpkin flesh with the other ingredients, simmer for 5 minutes, divide into cups and serve cold.

Nutrition:

Calories 192

Fat 3.4 Fiber 4.5

Carbs 7.6

Protein 3.5

Minty Coconut Cream

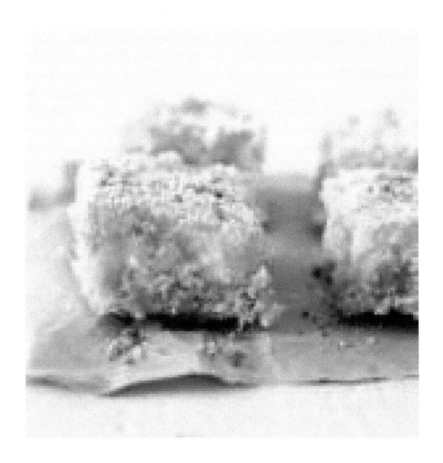

Preparation Time: 4 minutes

Cooking Time: 0 minutes

Servings: 2

Ingredients:

1 banana, peeled

2 cups coconut flesh, shredded

3 tablespoons mint, chopped

1 and ½ cups coconut water

2 tablespoons stevia

½ avocado, pitted and peeled

Directions:

In a blender, combine the coconut with the banana and the rest of the ingredients, pulse well, divide into cups and serve cold.

Nutrition:

Calories 193

Fat 5.4

Fiber 3.4

Carbs 7.6

Protein 3

Watermelon Cream

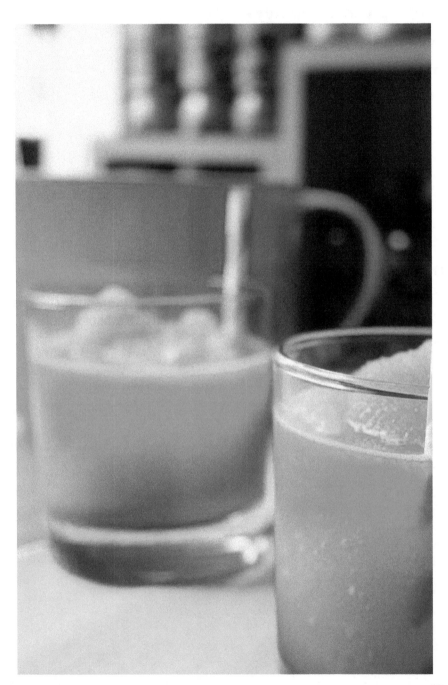

Preparation Time: 15 minutes

Cooking Time: 0 minutes

Servings: 2

Ingredients:

1 pound watermelon, peeled and chopped

1 teaspoon vanilla extract

1 cup heavy cream

1 teaspoon lime juice

2 tablespoons stevia

Directions:

In a blender, combine the watermelon with the cream and the rest of the ingredients, pulse well, divide into cups and keep in the fridge for 15 minutes before serving.

Nutrition:

Calories 122

Fat 5.7

Fiber 3.2

Carbs 5.3

Protein 0.4

Grapes Stew

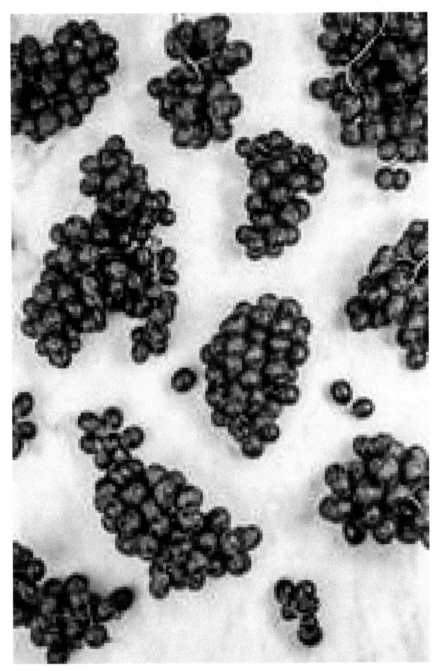

Preparation Time: 10 minutes

Cooking Time: 10 minutes

Servings: 4

Ingredients:

2/3 cup stevia

1 tablespoon olive oil

1/3 cup coconut water

1 teaspoon vanilla extract

1 teaspoon lemon zest, grated

2 cup red grapes, halved

Directions:

Heat up a pan with the water over medium heat, add the oil, stevia and the rest of the ingredients, toss, simmer for 10 minutes, divide into cups and serve.

Nutrition:

Calories 122

Fat 3.7

Fiber 1.2

Carbs 2.3

Protein 0.4

Strawberry Muffins

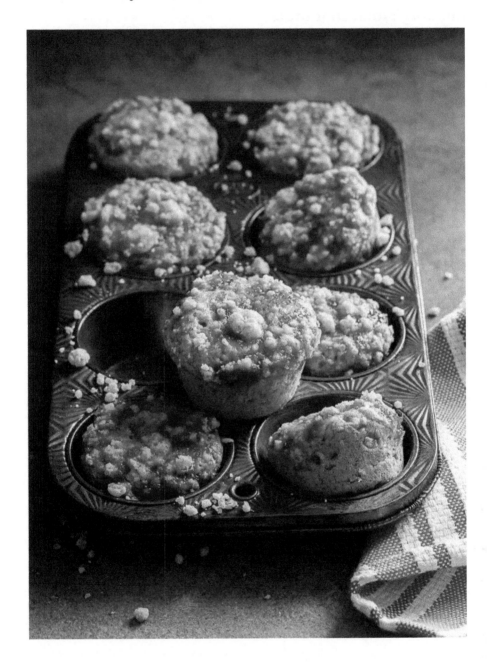

Difficulty Level: 2/5

Preparation time: 5 minutes

Cooking time: 25 minutes

Servings:: 8

Ingredients

2 cup Wheat flour

1 cup Strawberry

1/2 cup Milk

2 fl. oz Olive oil

1 Egg

2 tsp Baking powder

Sugar and salt, to taste

Directions:

In a bowl, mix the baking powder, sugar, and flour. In another bowl, beat the egg with milk and olive oil.

Mix both mixtures and mix well. Add a glass of sliced strawberries and mix gently, without damaging the berries.

Grease the muffin pan with butter or put a paper mold in each hole. Fill two-thirds doughs and bake for 20-25 minutes in an oven preheated to 375 degrees until cooked.

Allow to cool in shape, then shift to a platter.

Nutrition: (Per serving)

Calories: 284 Kcal

Fat: 8 g.

Protein: 5.3 g.

Carbs: 48 g.

Compote Dipped Berries Mix

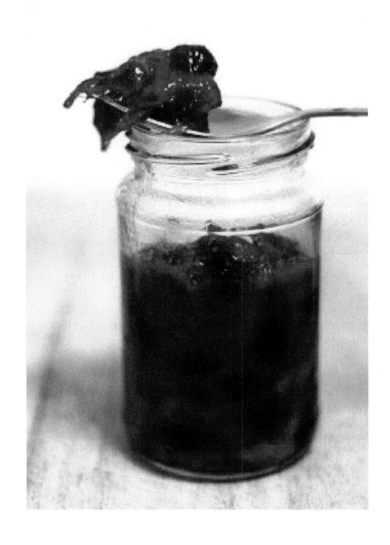

Preparation Time: 10 minutes

Cooking time: 10 minutes

Servings: 8

Ingredients:

2 cups fresh strawberries, hulled and halved lengthwise

4 sprigs fresh mint

2 cups fresh blackberries

1 cup pomegranate juice

2 teaspoons vanilla

6 orange pekoe tea bags

2 cups fresh red raspberries

1 cup water

2 cups fresh golden raspberries

2 cups fresh sweet cherries, pitted and halved

2 cups fresh blueberries

2 ml bottle Sauvignon Blanc

Directions:

Preheat the oven to 290 degrees F and lightly grease a baking dish.

Soak mint sprigs and tea bags in boiled water for about 10 minutes in a covered bowl.

Mix together all the berries and cherries in another bowl and keep aside.

Cook wine with pomegranate juice in a saucepan and add strained tea liquid.

Toss in the mixed berries to serve and enjoy.

Nutrition:

Calories 356

Total Fat 0.8 g

Saturated Fat 0.1 g

Cholesterol 0 mg

Total Carbs 89.9 g

Dietary Fiber 9.4 g

Sugar 70.8 g

Protein 2.2 g

Popped Quinoa Bars

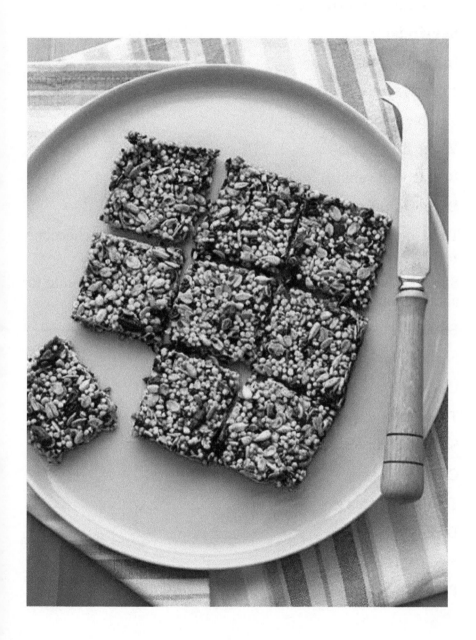

Preparation Time: 10 minutes

Cooking time: 10 minutes

Servings: 3

Ingredients:

2 (4 oz.) semi-sweet chocolate bars, chopped

½ tablespoon peanut butter

½ cup dry quinoa

¼ teaspoon vanilla

Directions:

Toast dry quinoa in a pan until golden and stir in chocolate, vanilla and peanut butter.

Spread this mixture in a baking sheet evenly and refrigerate for about 4 hours.

Break it into small pieces and serve chilled.

Nutrition:

Calories 278

Total Fat 11.8 g

Saturated Fat 6.6 g

Cholesterol 7 mg

Total Carbs 36.2 g

Dietary Fiber 3.1 g

Sugar 15.4 g

Protein 6.9 g

Almond Orange Pandoro

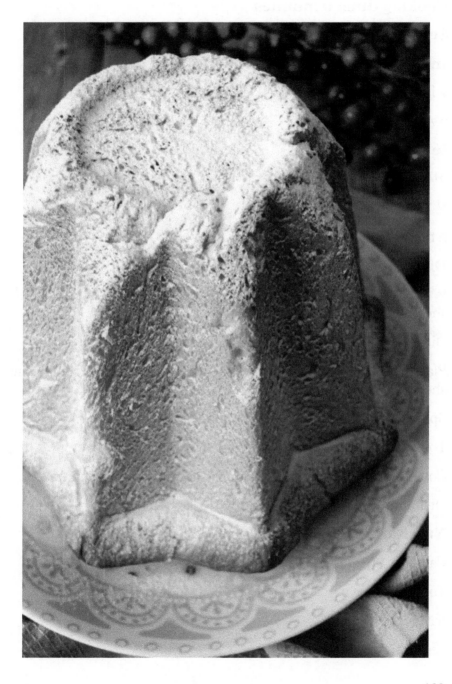

Preparation Time: 10 minutes

Cooking time: 0 minutes

Servings: 12

Ingredients:

2 large oranges, zested

2½ cups mascarpone

½ cup almonds, whole

2½ cups coconut cream

½ pandoro, diced

2 tablespoons sherry

Directions:

Whisk cream with mascarpone, icing sugar, ¾ zest and half sherry in a bowl.

Dice the pandoro into equal sized horizontal slices.

Place the bottom slice in a plate and top with the remaining sherry.

Spoon the mascarpone mixture over the slice.

Top with almonds and place another pandoro slice over.

Continue adding layers of pandoro slices and cream mixture.

Dish out to serve.

Nutrition:

Calories 346

Total Fat 10.4 g

Saturated Fat 3 g

Cholesterol 10 mg

Total Carbs 8.5 g

Dietary Fiber 3 g

Sugar 2.4 g

Protein 7.7 g

Mango-Pear Smoothie

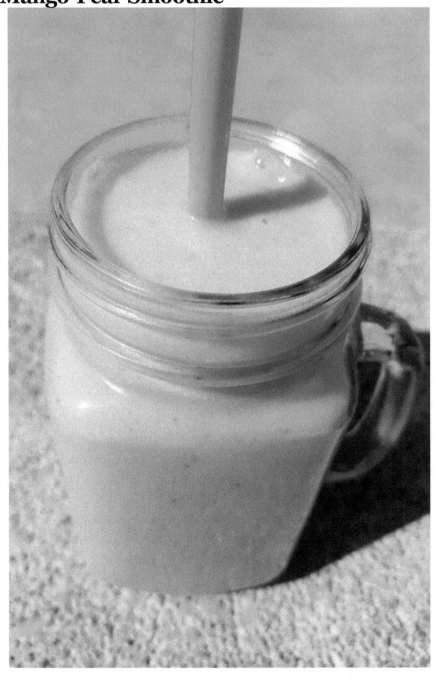

Difficulty Level: 1/5

Preparation time: 10 minutes

Cooking time: 0 minutes

Servings: 1

Ingredients:

1 ripe pear, cored and chopped

½ mango, peeled, pitted, and chopped

1 cup chopped kale

½ cup plain Greek yogurt

2 ice cubes

Directions:

In a blender, purée the pear, mango, kale, and yogurt.

Add the ice and blend until thick and smooth. Pour the smoothie into a glass and serve cold.

Nutrition:

Calories: 293;

Total Fat: 8g;

Saturated Fat: 5g;

Carbohydrates: 53g;

Fiber: 7g;

Protein: 8g

Strawberry-Rhubarb Smoothie
Difficulty Level: 2/5

Preparation time: 5 minutes

Cooking time: 3 minutes

Servings: 1

Ingredients:

1 rhubarb stalk, chopped

1 cup sliced fresh strawberries

½ cup plain Greek yogurt

2 tablespoons honey

Pinch ground cinnamon

3 ice cubes

Directions:

Place a small saucepan filled with water over high heat and bring to a boil. Add the rhubarb and boil for 3 minutes. Drain and transfer the rhubarb to a blender.

Add the strawberries, yogurt, honey, and cinnamon and pulse the mixture until it is smooth.

Add the ice and blend until thick, with no ice lumps remaining. Pour the smoothie into a glass and enjoy cold.

Nutrition:

Calories: 295;

Total Fat: 8g;

Saturated Fat: 5g;

Carbohydrates: 56g;

Fiber: 4g;

Protein: 6g

Lightning Source UK Ltd.
Milton Keynes UK
UKHW020657310521
384668UK00001B/84

9 781802 697544